THE WAY OF THE ETERNAL ISLE: UNLOCKING THE OKINAWA SECRET

DIPAN KUMAR DAS

SUDIP KUMAR DAS

To all those who have walked the shores of Okinawa, who have listened to the whispers of its winds, and who have been touched by the wisdom of its people.

This book is dedicated to the Okinawans, whose vibrant spirits and deep-rooted traditions have inspired generations. Your commitment to health, longevity, and the pursuit of happiness is a beacon of light in a world filled with challenges.

We also dedicate this book to the readers, the seekers of knowledge and inspiration. May the wisdom shared within these pages ignite a spark within you, guiding you on a transformative journey towards a healthier, happier, and more fulfilling life.

To the researchers, scientists, and scholars who tirelessly unravel the secrets behind Okinawa's exceptional longevity, we honor your dedication to uncovering the science behind the magic.

To the elders of Okinawa, the guardians of ancient wisdom, we express our deepest gratitude for sharing your stories, your traditions, and your precious knowledge with the world.

To the future generations, may you carry the spirit of Okinawa forward, embracing its wisdom, and nurturing the eternal isle within yourselves and the world around you.

Finally, we dedicate this book to the interconnectedness of all living beings. May we recognize our shared humanity, our shared pursuit of health and happiness, and work together to create a world where the secrets of Okinawa are celebrated and applied for the well-being of all.

This book is dedicated with love, respect, and gratitude to all who have contributed to the preservation and dissemination of the Okinawa secret.

Foreword

In the vast ocean of self-help books and wellness literature, there are few gems that truly stand out, offering profound insights and guiding readers towards a life of vitality and purpose. "The Okinawa Secret" is undoubtedly one of those rare gems.

As I had the privilege of reading through the pages of this remarkable book, I was captivated by the rich tapestry of Okinawan wisdom and the lessons it holds for all of humanity. The Okinawa

Secret is not just about living longer; it is about living better, with a deep sense of purpose, joy, and connection.

In this book, the authors take us on a captivating journey to the enchanting island of Okinawa, where the inhabitants defy the odds of aging and embrace life with a remarkable vigor. Through careful research, interviews, and personal anecdotes, they unravel the secrets behind Okinawa's exceptional longevity and offer practical insights on how to apply these principles to our own lives.

What makes "The Okinawa Secret" truly remarkable is its holistic approach. It recognizes that longevity and well-being are not solely determined by diet or exercise but are the result of a harmonious interplay between various aspects of life. From the Okinawan diet to physical activity, from nurturing body and mind to finding purpose and meaning, every chapter explores a key element of the Okinawa secret, weaving them together into a tapestry of wisdom and guidance.

But this book is not merely a collection of facts and advice; it is an invitation to reflect, to question our own beliefs and lifestyle choices, and to embark on a transformative journey towards a healthier and more fulfilling life. It challenges us to reassess our priorities, to embrace change, and to cultivate a mindset that nurtures our well-being and that of those around us.

As I immersed myself in the pages of "The Okinawa Secret," I found myself inspired and motivated to make positive changes in my own life. The stories of Okinawans living vibrant and purposeful lives well into their centenarian years serve as a testament to the power of embracing the Okinawa secret.

I am grateful to the authors for bringing this extraordinary wisdom to light and sharing it with the world. Their passion for the subject matter is evident in every word, and their commitment to honoring the traditions and teachings of Okinawa shines through.

I invite you, dear reader, to embark on this transformative journey with an open heart and mind. Allow the wisdom of Okinawa to seep into your being, guiding you towards a life filled with vitality, purpose, and joy. Embrace the Okinawa secret and unlock the eternal isle within.

Preface

It is with great pleasure and excitement that we present to you "The Okinawa Secret." This book is the culmination of our deep fascination with the extraordinary longevity and well-being of the people of Okinawa, an island in Japan that has captured the world's attention.

As we embarked on this journey of exploration, we were drawn to the enigmatic allure surrounding the Okinawa secret. The stories of Okinawans living healthy and fulfilling lives well into their 100s sparked our curiosity and ignited a desire to understand the underlying principles behind their exceptional longevity.

Our quest took us on a voyage to the enchanting shores of Okinawa, where we had the privilege of immersing ourselves in its vibrant culture, connecting with its people, and delving into the treasure trove of wisdom that has been passed down through generations.

Through countless interviews, discussions with experts, and deep dives into scientific research, we unraveled the layers of the Okinawa secret. What we discovered was a holistic tapestry of principles and practices that go far beyond diet and exercise. It encompasses a profound connection to nature, a sense of purpose and meaning, strong social bonds, and a harmonious balance of body, mind, and spirit.

In this book, we aim to share with you the essence of the Okinawa secret, distilling its wisdom into practical guidance that can be integrated into your own life. We delve into the traditional

Okinawan diet, explore the importance of physical activity and mental well-being, uncover the concept of ikigai (purpose), and discuss strategies for stress reduction and maintaining balance.

But "The Okinawa Secret" is not just a compilation of information. It is an invitation to embark on a transformative journey towards a healthier, happier, and more fulfilling life. It encourages you to question your own beliefs and lifestyle choices, to embrace change, and to cultivate a mindset that supports your well-being and vitality.

We hope that the stories, insights, and practical tips shared within these pages inspire you to adopt the principles of the Okinawa secret and make positive changes in your life. May this book be a guiding light, illuminating your path towards enhanced health, longevity, and a deeper sense of purpose.

We express our deepest gratitude to the people of Okinawa, whose warmth, wisdom, and generosity have enriched our lives and the lives of countless others. We also extend our appreciation to the researchers, experts, and scholars who have dedicated their efforts to unraveling the mysteries of Okinawa's exceptional well-being.

We invite you to open your heart and mind as you embark on this journey with us. Embrace the Okinawa secret and unlock the eternal isle within yourself.

Prologue

In the vast expanse of the Pacific Ocean lies a hidden gem, a place where time seems to move at a different pace and where the secrets of longevity and well-being are whispered by the winds. This place is Okinawa, an island that holds the key to a remarkable mystery—the Okinawa secret.

For centuries, Okinawa has captivated the hearts and minds of explorers, researchers, and seekers of wisdom. Its inhabitants, known for their exceptional health and vitality, have puzzled scientists and sparked a global fascination with their ability to live long and fulfilling lives.

As we step into the realm of Okinawa, we are transported to a world where age is revered, where the wisdom of the elders is cherished, and where the rhythm of life beats in harmony with nature. Here, the air is infused with a sense of tranquility, and the land bears the imprints of a resilient culture shaped by centuries of history and tradition.

But what is it that sets Okinawa apart? What is the secret to the longevity and well-being of its people? Is it simply the result of genetics, or is there something more profound at play?

In the pages that follow, we invite you to join us on a journey of discovery—a journey that will unravel the Okinawa secret and illuminate the path to a healthier, happier, and more purposeful existence. We will delve into the depths of Okinawan culture, explore the science behind its exceptional longevity, and uncover the timeless wisdom that holds the key to a life of vitality and fulfillment.

Prepare to be inspired by the stories of centenarians who defy the limitations of age and embrace life with zest. Marvel at the power of the Okinawan diet, a culinary tapestry woven with nutritious ingredients that nourish both body and soul. Explore the profound connection between physical activity, mental well-being, and longevity as we delve into the practices that keep Okinawans vibrant and resilient.

But the Okinawa secret is not confined to the physical realm alone. It encompasses a deeper understanding of purpose and meaning, the cultivation of strong social connections, and the ability to find balance and harmony in a fast-paced world. It is a holistic approach to life that touches every aspect of our being.

As we embark on this journey together, let us open our hearts and minds to the wisdom of Okinawa. Let us embrace the lessons it offers and integrate its principles into our own lives. For within the Okinawa secret lies a profound truth—that by nourishing our bodies, nurturing our spirits, and finding our own sense of purpose, we too can unlock the eternal isle within ourselves.

The time has come to unveil the mysteries of Okinawa, to embrace its wisdom, and to embark on a transformative journey towards a life of health, longevity, and fulfillment. Let us step into the realm of the Okinawa secret and unlock its hidden treasures.

Welcome to "The Okinawa Secret."

CHAPTER ONE
Introduction to Okinawa

Nestled in the azure waters of the East China Sea lies Okinawa, a captivating Japanese island renowned for its extraordinary longevity and vibrant population of centenarians. For decades, researchers and health enthusiasts alike have been captivated by the "Okinawa secret" – the enigmatic factors that contribute to the islanders' exceptional health, longevity, and remarkable quality of life. In this book, "The Way of the Eternal Isle: Unlocking the Okinawa Secret," we embark on a captivating journey to unravel the mysteries behind Okinawa's unique demographics and explore the fascinating facets of its time-honored lifestyle.

Okinawa's demographics present an intriguing phenomenon. This idyllic island boasts one of the highest concentrations of centenarians in the world, with an abundance of vibrant individuals who have surpassed the age of 100. It is not uncommon to encounter elders who exude vitality, engage in active lifestyles, and possess remarkable physical and cognitive abilities well into their golden years. Researchers have pondered over the factors that contribute to Okinawa's longevity for decades, leading to a widespread fascination and a yearning to uncover the secrets that lie within its shores.

In this brief overview, we will delve into Okinawa's unique demographics and longevity statistics, providing a glimpse into the striking numbers that have astounded researchers and inspired countless individuals seeking to unlock the keys to a long and healthy life. We will explore the intriguing question: What sets Okinawa apart from other regions, and how can we harness the lessons learned from this island paradise to enhance our own well-being?

Beyond the captivating statistics, the allure of Okinawa's longevity secret extends to the rich cultural heritage and the inherent wisdom passed down through generations. Throughout this journey, we will explore the island's traditions, rituals, and lifestyle practices that have played an integral role in shaping the health and vitality of its inhabitants. From the renowned Okinawan diet to the profound sense of purpose and community connections, each facet of Okinawan life holds valuable insights that can empower us to lead healthier, more fulfilling lives.

As we embark on this exploration of the Okinawa secret, it is important to approach it with an open mind and a genuine curiosity. While we may not discover a single magical elixir or a quick-fix solution, we will unveil a holistic approach to well-being that encompasses the mind, body, and spirit. The Okinawa secret encompasses more than just nutrition or exercise; it is a way of life that embraces balance, purpose, and interconnectedness with nature and community.

"The Way of the Eternal Isle: Unlocking the Okinawa Secret" is an invitation to embark on a transformative journey that transcends boundaries and taps into the timeless wisdom of Okinawa. Prepare to immerse yourself in the depths of Okinawan culture, learn from its elders, and adopt practical strategies that can enhance your longevity, vitality, and overall well-being. Together, let us unravel the Okinawa secret and discover the path to a fulfilling and enduring life.

In our quest to unlock the Okinawa secret, we will draw upon a wealth of scientific research, personal anecdotes, and cultural insights. We will examine the pillars of Okinawan life that contribute to their remarkable health and longevity, and we will uncover practical ways to integrate these principles into our own lives.

One of the key aspects we will explore is the Okinawan diet, a cornerstone of their lifestyle. We will delve into the specific foods that form the foundation of their meals, such as nutrient-rich vegetables, fruits, whole grains, and legumes. We will discover the powerful health benefits of their dietary choices, including reduced risks of chronic diseases like heart disease, cancer, and diabetes. By understanding the principles behind the Okinawan diet, we can make informed decisions about our own nutrition and create a more balanced and nourishing approach to eating.

Beyond the realm of nutrition, we will uncover the significance of an active lifestyle in Okinawan culture. We will explore the various physical activities that Okinawans engage in throughout their lives, from traditional martial arts like karate and tai chi to daily practices such as walking and gardening. By embracing the Okinawan approach to physical activity, we can enhance our physical fitness, improve our mental well-being, and cultivate a sense of purpose and fulfillment in our daily lives.

Moreover, we will delve into the concept of ikigai, a central theme in Okinawan philosophy. Ikigai represents the intersection of one's passions, talents, and sense of purpose. We will explore how Okinawans discover and nurture their ikigai, and we will learn practical strategies to uncover our own life's purpose. By aligning our actions and goals with our sense of ikigai, we can experience a deeper sense of meaning and fulfillment, leading to a more vibrant and purpose-driven existence.

Stress reduction and the cultivation of inner peace will also be explored. We will examine the stress management techniques practiced by Okinawans, including meditation, mindfulness, and time spent in nature. We will learn how to incorporate these practices into our lives to promote mental clarity, reduce stress, and foster a sense of balance and well-being.

Throughout our journey, we will highlight the profound connection between Okinawans and their natural environment. Okinawa's breathtaking landscapes, mild climate, and proximity to the ocean have a profound impact on the well-being of its inhabitants. We will discover the therapeutic benefits of immersing ourselves in nature, engaging in outdoor activities, and embracing the serenity and beauty that surrounds us.

"The Way of the Eternal Isle: Unlocking the Okinawa Secret" is an invitation to explore a way of life that transcends age-old wisdom and scientific discoveries. By embracing the principles and practices of Okinawa, we can embark on a transformative path toward improved health, longevity, and fulfillment. So, join us as we unveil the Okinawa secret and embark on a journey toward a vibrant and enduring life, inspired by the wisdom of the Eternal Isle.

In the final chapters of our book, "The Way of the Eternal Isle: Unlocking the Okinawa Secret," we will bring together the knowledge and insights gained from our exploration of Okinawan culture, nutrition, physical activity, purpose, stress reduction, and connection to nature. We will provide practical guidance on how to incorporate these principles into our everyday lives and create a holistic approach to well-being.

Through actionable steps and tips, we will empower readers to make positive changes in their diets by adopting Okinawan-inspired meal plans and recipes that prioritize nutrient-dense, plant-based foods. We will offer guidance on sourcing and preparing these ingredients, making it easier to integrate the Okinawan diet into our own culinary practices.

Furthermore, we will delve into the practical aspects of incorporating physical activity into our routines. Whether it's through engaging in martial arts, practicing mindful movement, or simply adding more movement into our daily lives, we will provide actionable strategies to help readers cultivate an active and vibrant lifestyle.

Understanding the significance of purpose in our lives, we will guide readers in discovering their own ikigai. Through reflection exercises, guidance on exploring passions and talents, and creating meaningful goals, we will assist readers in aligning their actions with their sense of purpose and finding greater fulfillment in their endeavors.

Stress reduction and finding balance will be addressed with practical techniques that can be easily integrated into daily routines. We will provide guidance on various relaxation methods, meditation practices, and strategies for managing time and priorities effectively. By implementing these stress-reducing techniques, readers can create a more peaceful and harmonious existence, improving their overall well-being.

Finally, we will explore ways to deepen our connection with nature, even in urban environments. By highlighting the benefits of spending time outdoors, engaging in nature-based activities, and fostering a sense of awe and gratitude for the natural world, readers will discover ways to incorporate the healing power of nature into their lives.

As we conclude our journey, we will emphasize that the Okinawa secret is not a quick-fix solution or a one-size-fits-all approach. It is a holistic way of life that encompasses multiple facets of well-being. By embracing the principles and practices inspired by Okinawa, readers can create their own unique path to enhanced health, longevity, and fulfillment.

"The Way of the Eternal Isle: Unlocking the Okinawa Secret" will equip readers with the knowledge, inspiration, and practical tools to embark on their own transformative journey. By integrating the wisdom of Okinawa into their lives, readers can experience profound changes that lead to a vibrant, enduring, and purposeful existence.

So, let us embark together on this captivating exploration, immersing ourselves in the Okinawa secret and discovering the path to a life of health, longevity, and fulfillment. The Eternal Isle awaits, ready to share its secrets and wisdom with those who are willing to embrace its timeless teachings.

CHAPTER TWO

The Okinawan Diet: Nourishing Body and Mind

Introduction: In this chapter, we will embark on a journey into the heart of Okinawa's famed diet. We will delve into the rich tapestry of ingredients, culinary traditions, and nutritional principles that form the foundation of the Okinawan way of eating. By understanding the key components of the Okinawan diet and the science behind its positive effects, we can unlock the secrets to longevity and overall well-being.

Key Components of the Okinawan Diet: We will explore the key components that make the Okinawan diet unique and health-promoting. This includes an abundance of fresh fruits and vegetables, whole grains, legumes, soy products, seafood, and seaweed. We will delve into the nutritional properties of these foods and how they contribute to the overall health and vitality of Okinawans.

The Okinawan Caloric Restriction: One of the remarkable aspects of the Okinawan diet is its caloric restriction. Okinawans traditionally consume fewer calories compared to many other populations, while still meeting their nutritional needs. We will examine the science behind caloric restriction and its potential benefits for longevity and disease prevention. Additionally, we will discuss practical strategies for implementing mindful eating and portion control in our own lives.

Nutritional Powerhouses and Antioxidants: Certain foods and ingredients play a significant role in the Okinawan diet's health benefits. We will highlight nutritional powerhouses like purple sweet potatoes, bitter melon, turmeric, and green tea, which are rich in antioxidants and have been associated with various health benefits. We will delve into the science behind these antioxidants, their impact on cellular health, and how they contribute to Okinawans' overall well-being.

Gut Health and Fermented Foods: Fermented foods are a prominent feature of the Okinawan diet. We will explore the importance of gut health and the role of fermented foods such as miso, tofu, natto, and pickled vegetables in promoting a healthy microbiome. We will discuss the benefits of probiotics, prebiotics, and their potential effects on immune function, digestion, and overall well-being.

Balanced Nutrition and Longevity: The Okinawan diet emphasizes a balanced approach to nutrition, with an abundance of plant-based foods, moderate amounts of fish and seafood, and limited consumption of meat and dairy. We will discuss the science behind this balance and explore how it contributes to reduced risks of chronic diseases, such as heart disease, certain cancers, and age-related conditions.

Beyond Food: Mindful Eating and Social Connections: The Okinawan diet goes beyond the food itself; it encompasses the cultural and social aspects of eating. We will explore the importance of mindful eating, savoring each bite, and fostering a positive relationship with food. Additionally, we will examine the Okinawan tradition of communal meals, where shared dining experiences and strong social connections contribute to overall well-being.

Practical Tips and Recipes: To help readers integrate the Okinawan diet into their own lives, we will provide practical tips for grocery shopping, meal planning, and preparation. We will share simple and delicious Okinawan-inspired recipes that showcase the flavors and health benefits of this traditional way of eating.

As we conclude our exploration of the Okinawan diet, we will reflect on the profound impact of nutrition on longevity and overall well-being. By adopting the principles of the Okinawan diet, we can nourish our bodies, cultivate balance, and unlock the potential for a vibrant and enduring life.

Exploring Okinawan Food Culture: In this section, we will delve into the unique food culture of Okinawa and its impact on the Okinawan diet. We will explore the historical influences and cultural practices that have shaped Okinawan cuisine, such as the use of local ingredients, traditional cooking methods, and the incorporation of flavors from neighboring East Asian countries. Understanding the cultural context of the Okinawan diet will deepen our appreciation for its significance and provide insights into its health-promoting aspects.

Science Behind the Okinawan Diet: To truly comprehend the impact of the

Okinawan diet on longevity and well-being, we will explore the scientific research and studies conducted on Okinawan populations. We will examine the findings related to reduced risks of chronic diseases, improved markers of cardiovascular health, enhanced cognitive function, and overall longevity. By understanding the scientific basis of the Okinawan diet, we can better appreciate its potential benefits for our own health.

Environmental and Sustainability Considerations: As we embrace the Okinawan diet, it is crucial to consider its environmental and sustainability implications. We will discuss the importance of sourcing local, seasonal, and organic foods to reduce our carbon footprint and support sustainable agricultural practices. Exploring the

Okinawan principles of minimal waste and reverence for nature, we will discover how our dietary choices can contribute to a more sustainable future.

Adapting the Okinawan Diet to Modern Lifestyles: While staying true to the essence of the Okinawan diet, we recognize that adapting it to modern lifestyles may be necessary. In this section, we will provide practical guidance on how to incorporate the principles of the Okinawan diet into our own daily lives, taking into account diverse dietary preferences, cultural considerations, and practical constraints. Whether it involves modifying recipes, sourcing local ingredients, or finding alternatives, we will explore strategies to make the Okinawan diet accessible and sustainable for everyone.

Beyond Nutrition: Okinawan Mindset and Well-being: The Okinawan diet is not solely about food; it is a reflection of a broader mindset and approach to life. In this final section, we will explore the connection between the Okinawan diet and overall well-being. We will discuss the importance of cultivating a positive mindset, embracing a sense of gratitude, finding joy in simple pleasures, and maintaining strong social connections. Understanding the holistic nature of the Okinawan lifestyle will empower us to not only adopt their dietary practices but also embody their broader approach to wellness.

As we conclude our exploration of the Okinawan diet, we will reflect on the transformative power of nourishing our bodies and minds through the principles of this time-honored way of eating. By embracing the richness of Okinawan cuisine, integrating its nutritional wisdom, and adopting its holistic mindset, we can unlock the potential for a healthier, more fulfilling life. The Okinawan diet invites us to savor each bite, honor the connection between food and well-being, and embark on a journey towards longevity, vitality, and inner balance.

Promoting Longevity and Disease Prevention: In this section, we will delve deeper into the specific health benefits associated with the Okinawan diet. We will explore the research linking the Okinawan diet to longevity and disease prevention. From lower rates of heart disease and stroke to a reduced risk of age-related conditions like dementia, we will examine the scientific evidence that supports the positive impact of the

Okinawan diet on overall health and well-being.

Understanding Macronutrient Balance: A critical aspect of the Okinawan diet is its unique macronutrient balance. We will explore the traditional ratios of carbohydrates, proteins, and fats in the Okinawan diet and discuss the potential benefits of this balance for metabolic health, weight management, and sustained energy levels. We will also consider the quality of macronutrients consumed, highlighting the importance of choosing whole, unprocessed sources for optimal nutrition.

Exploring Culinary Techniques and Flavor Profiles: Okinawan cuisine is not only about the ingredients but also the cooking techniques and flavor profiles that make it distinctive. We will uncover the cooking methods employed in

Okinawan dishes, such as stir-frying, steaming, and simmering, which help retain the nutritional integrity of the foods. We will also explore the unique flavors and seasonings used in Okinawan cooking, including island spices, herbs, and locally sourced ingredients, which contribute to both taste and health benefits.

Seasonality and Locally Sourced Foods: The Okinawan diet emphasizes the importance of seasonality and locally sourced foods. We will delve into the significance of consuming foods that are in harmony with the natural rhythm of the environment and discuss the benefits of supporting local farmers and food producers. By prioritizing seasonal and locally sourced foods, we can enhance the freshness, nutritional value, and sustainability of our diets.

The Role of Okinawan Tea: Tea holds a special place in Okinawan culture and is a staple in the Okinawan diet. We will explore the different types of Okinawan tea, such as jasmine tea and the unique herbal infusion called sanpin-cha. We will uncover the health benefits associated with tea consumption, including its antioxidant properties, potential effects on weight management, and its role in promoting relaxation and mental well-being.

Okinawan Diet in a Modern Context: As we navigate the modern world, we will address the challenges and opportunities of adopting the Okinawan diet. We will provide practical tips for incorporating Okinawan-inspired meals into busy lifestyles, including meal planning, batch cooking, and making informed choices when dining out. We will also explore how technology and online resources can support our journey toward embracing the Okinawan diet and lifestyle.

Conclusion: As we conclude our exploration of the Okinawan diet, we will reflect on the remarkable synergy between nutrition, culture, and well-being. The Okinawan diet offers us not only a blueprint for nourishing our bodies but also a path to cultivating balance, connection, and longevity. By embracing the principles of the Okinawan diet, we can embark on a transformative journey toward optimal health, enhanced vitality, and a deep appreciation for the interplay between food, culture, and well-being.

CHAPTER THREE

Nurturing Body and Mind: The Essence of Physical Activity and Mental Well-being in Okinawan Culture

Introduction: In this chapter, we will explore the integral role of physical activity and mental well-being in the lives of Okinawans. We will delve into the rich tapestry of activities, practices, and traditions that contribute to the overall health, vitality, and longevity of the Okinawan people. By understanding the importance of nurturing both the body and mind, we can gain insights into the Okinawan approach to holistic well-being.

Martial Arts: The Way of Self-Defense and Discipline: Martial arts have deep roots in Okinawan culture and have been practiced for centuries. We will explore the significance of martial arts, such as karate, kobudo, and Okinawan sumo, in promoting physical strength, discipline, and mental focus. We will delve into the principles and philosophies underlying these martial arts, and how they contribute to the overall well-being and character development of practitioners.

Dance and Music: Expressions of Joy and Cultural Identity: Traditional Okinawan dance and music are not only artistic expressions but also forms of physical activity that promote vitality and emotional well-being. We will discover the various dance forms, such as the energetic Eisa dance and the graceful Ryukyu court dances, and their connection to Okinawan culture and identity. We will also explore the health benefits of dance, including improved coordination, cardiovascular fitness, and the release of endorphins that enhance mood and overall well-being.

Gardening: Cultivating Connection with Nature and Physical Engagement: Okinawans have a strong affinity for gardening, which goes beyond the act of growing plants. We will uncover the therapeutic aspects of gardening, such as connecting with nature, physical activity, and the sense of accomplishment derived from nurturing plants. We will discuss the practice of tsubo-niwa (courtyard gardening) and how it promotes relaxation, stress reduction, and a sense of purpose and fulfillment.

Mindfulness and Meditation: Cultivating Inner Balance and Mental Resilience: Okinawans embrace mindfulness and meditation as essential practices for mental well-being. We will explore various mindfulness techniques, including breathing exercises, mindful walking, and Zen meditation, and their positive effects on reducing stress, increasing self-awareness, and promoting mental resilience. We will delve into the role of mindfulness in Okinawan daily life and how it contributes to their overall sense of calm and equanimity.

Connection to Nature: Embracing the Healing Power of the Outdoors: Okinawans have a deep connection with nature, and spending time outdoors is an integral part of their lifestyle. We will discuss the benefits of nature immersion, such as forest bathing (shinrin-yoku), beach activities, and connecting with the ocean. We will explore the restorative effects of being in nature, including reduced stress, improved mood, and enhanced overall well-being.

Holistic Approaches to Well-being: Integrating Physical and Mental Practices: In this section, we will explore the interconnectedness of physical activity and mental well-being in the Okinawan approach to holistic health. We will discuss the integration of physical and mental practices, such as combining mindfulness with physical activities like tai chi or yoga. We will explore how these integrated practices contribute to overall balance, vitality, and a sense of inner harmony.

Practical Tips and Guidance: To help readers incorporate the Okinawan practices of physical activity and mental well-being into their own lives, we will provide practical tips and guidance. From finding local martial arts or dance classes to establishing a home meditation practice or creating a small garden space, we will offer actionable steps to cultivate a lifestyle that nurtures both the body and mind.

As we conclude our exploration of physical activity

and mental well-being in Okinawan culture, we are reminded of the profound connection between the body, mind, and overall health. The Okinawan people have embraced a holistic approach to well-being, recognizing the importance of nurturing both physical and mental aspects of their lives. By immersing ourselves in the practices and traditions that have sustained the Okinawans for generations, we can unlock the potential for enhanced vitality, resilience, and a deeper sense of fulfillment.

Embracing Physical Activity as a Lifestyle: Physical activity is not seen as a chore or a separate entity in Okinawan culture; rather, it is woven seamlessly into daily life. We will explore how Okinawans incorporate movement through activities like walking, cycling, and engaging in outdoor pursuits. We will highlight the benefits of adopting a lifestyle that prioritizes regular physical activity and the positive impact it has on cardiovascular health, muscle strength, bone density, and overall longevity.

The Role of Social Connections: Okinawans understand the importance of social connections in promoting well-being. We will examine the strong community bonds that exist within Okinawan society and how they contribute to mental and emotional health. We will discuss the concept of "moai," a close-knit social support network that provides a sense of belonging, companionship, and emotional support. We will explore how fostering meaningful connections with others can positively impact our mental well-being and overall life satisfaction.

Cultivating Resilience and Inner Strength: The Okinawan people possess a remarkable resilience and inner strength, which enables them to navigate life's challenges with grace and optimism. We will delve into the mindset and practices that foster this resilience, including the concept of "ikigai" (finding purpose and meaning in life), the importance of self-reflection, and the practice of gratitude. We will explore how cultivating resilience and inner strength contributes to mental well-being and overall life satisfaction.

Harmonizing Body and Mind: In Okinawan culture, the body and mind are seen as interconnected, with each influencing the other. We will discuss the concept of "nuchi du takara" (life is a treasure), which emphasizes the holistic nature of well-being. We will explore how practices such as mindfulness, meditation, and breathwork help to harmonize the body and mind, reduce stress, enhance focus, and promote a sense of inner peace and balance.

Finding Joy in the Present Moment: The Okinawan people have a deep appreciation for the present moment and find joy in the simple pleasures of life. We will explore the concept of "yutori" (finding space and time), which encourages slowing down, savoring experiences, and being fully present. We will discuss how embracing mindfulness and cultivating a sense of yutori can enhance mental well-being, reduce anxiety, and foster a greater sense of contentment and happiness.

Continuing the Legacy: As we conclude our exploration of physical activity and mental well-being in Okinawan culture, we are inspired to carry forward the wisdom and practices of this remarkable community. By embracing a holistic approach to our own well-being, nurturing our bodies and minds, and fostering strong social connections, we can embark on a journey toward enhanced vitality, resilience, and a profound sense of inner well-being. The Okinawan legacy serves as a guiding light, reminding us that true health encompasses more than just the physical, and that by nurturing our bodies and minds, we can live vibrant, fulfilling lives.

CHAPTER FOUR

Ikigai: Discovering Purpose and Meaning in Life

Introduction: In this chapter, we will delve into the profound concept of ikigai, a key philosophy in Okinawan culture that has been attributed to their longevity and overall well-being. We will explore the meaning of ikigai, its significance in the lives of Okinawans, and how it can serve as a guiding principle for finding purpose and meaning in our own lives.

Unveiling the Essence of Ikigai: We will begin by unraveling the essence of ikigai, going beyond its literal translation of "reason for being." We will explore how ikigai encompasses a sense of purpose, passion, and fulfillment that arises from engaging in activities that align with our values, strengths, and interests. We will discuss the interconnectedness of ikigai with personal identity, well-being, and the pursuit of a meaningful life.

Okinawan Perspectives on Ikigai: Drawing from the wisdom of Okinawan elders and community members, we will gain insights into their perspectives on ikigai. We will explore how they discover and cultivate their ikigai throughout different stages of life, how it shapes their daily routines and decision-making, and the profound impact it has on their overall sense of happiness, contentment, and longevity.

Ikigai and Longevity: We will delve into the research and studies that have explored the connection between ikigai and longevity. We will examine how having a strong sense of purpose and meaning in life is associated with improved physical and mental health outcomes, reduced stress levels, and increased resilience. We will also discuss the role of ikigai in promoting a positive mindset, social connections, and a sense of belonging, all of which contribute to a longer and more fulfilling life.

Discovering Your Ikigai: In this section, we will provide practical guidance on how to uncover and nurture your own sense of ikigai. We will explore self-reflection exercises, introspective questions, and personal exploration techniques to help identify your passions, values, strengths, and interests. We will discuss the importance of aligning your work, relationships, and leisure activities with your ikigai to experience a greater sense of purpose and fulfillment.

Living in Alignment with Your Ikigai: Once you have discovered your ikigai, we will discuss practical strategies for incorporating it into your daily life. We will explore how to align your career, hobbies, relationships, and lifestyle choices with your ikigai, creating a harmonious and purpose-driven existence. We will also address the challenges and obstacles that may arise and provide guidance on overcoming them to live a more fulfilling and authentic life.

Cultivating a Sense of Ikigai in Community: We will explore the role of community in nurturing and sustaining ikigai. We will discuss the importance of surrounding yourself with like-minded individuals, building supportive relationships, and engaging in activities that foster a sense of belonging and shared purpose. We will also highlight the Okinawan tradition of "yuntaku" (meaningful conversations) and how it deepens connections and enriches the pursuit of ikigai.

Ikigai in Everyday Practices: To integrate ikigai into your daily life, we will provide practical tips and suggestions. From incorporating mindful rituals and self-care practices to pursuing hobbies and volunteering, we will explore how to infuse your daily routines with activities that align with your ikigai. We will also discuss the importance of embracing gratitude, resilience, and adaptability in your journey of living in alignment with your purpose.

As we conclude our exploration of ikigai, we are reminded of the transformative power of finding purpose and meaning in our lives. By embracing the Okinawan philosophy of ikigai, we can navigate our existence with a deeper

sense of fulfillment, contentment, and longevity. The concept of ikigai invites us to reflect on our passions, values, strengths, and interests, and to align our daily activities with our sense of purpose. By discovering and nurturing our ikigai, we can experience a profound shift in our perspective, leading to a more meaningful and fulfilling life.

As we journey toward uncovering our ikigai, it is essential to embrace self-reflection, introspection, and personal exploration. By asking ourselves meaningful questions, exploring our passions, and understanding our core values, we can begin to discern the activities and pursuits that bring us joy and a sense of purpose. Through this process, we can identify the unique combination of factors that make up our ikigai.

Living in alignment with our ikigai requires intentional choices and actions. It involves aligning our work, relationships, and leisure activities with our sense of purpose. By finding ways to incorporate our passions and interests into our careers or pursuing them as hobbies, we create a sense of harmony and fulfillment. Building supportive relationships and engaging in community activities that align with our ikigai also enhance our sense of belonging and contribute to our overall well-being.

Cultivating a sense of ikigai in our daily lives involves integrating it into our everyday practices. We can infuse our routines with mindful rituals, self-care practices, and activities that bring us joy and a sense of purpose. Embracing gratitude, resilience, and adaptability becomes paramount in navigating the challenges and obstacles that may arise along the way. By staying connected to our ikigai and continually nurturing it, we can lead a more authentic, purpose-driven life.

In the journey of discovering and embracing our ikigai, it is important to remember that it is a deeply personal and evolving process. Our ikigai may change and evolve as we grow and experience different stages of life. By remaining open to new possibilities and continually reassessing our passions, values, and interests, we can ensure that our pursuit of ikigai remains dynamic and fulfilling.

Ultimately, embracing the philosophy of ikigai allows us to tap into our innate potential, find deeper meaning in our lives, and experience a greater sense of happiness and well-being. By following the wisdom of the Okinawan people and integrating the concept of ikigai into our lives, we embark on a transformative journey that brings us closer to a life of purpose, fulfillment, and longevity.

Exploring Ikigai Across Cultures: While the concept of ikigai originated in Okinawan culture, its principles resonate with individuals across the globe. In this section, we will explore how ikigai can be understood and applied in different cultural contexts. We will examine how other cultures embrace the pursuit of purpose and meaning in life, and how their practices align with the essence of ikigai. By recognizing the universal nature of ikigai, we can draw inspiration from diverse perspectives and enrich our own understanding and pursuit of a meaningful life.

Overcoming Obstacles and Embracing Resilience: The journey of discovering and living in alignment with our ikigai is not without challenges. In this chapter, we will address common obstacles that may hinder our pursuit of purpose and offer strategies for overcoming them. We will explore how resilience, adaptability, and a growth mindset play crucial roles in navigating setbacks, doubts, and external pressures. By cultivating resilience and embracing challenges as opportunities for growth, we can continue moving forward on our path towards fulfilling our ikigai.

Passing Down the Legacy: The wisdom of ikigai has been passed down through generations, contributing to the longevity and well-being of the Okinawan people. In this section, we will discuss the importance of preserving and sharing the concept of ikigai with future generations. We will explore ways to incorporate ikigai in education, family life, and community initiatives, ensuring that its principles continue to inspire and guide individuals towards a life of purpose and meaning.

Conclusion: The concept of ikigai holds a profound significance in Okinawan culture, offering insights into the secret of their longevity and well-being. By uncovering our ikigai, we embark on a transformative journey towards a life of purpose, fulfillment, and vitality. Through self-reflection, intentional choices, and embracing challenges with resilience, we can align our actions and experiences with our deepest sense of meaning. By embracing the legacy of ikigai and sharing its wisdom, we contribute to a world where individuals lead purpose-driven lives, creating a ripple effect of positivity and well-being in ourselves and those around us. As we embrace the essence of ikigai, we tap into the infinite possibilities that await us on our journey towards a life of purpose, joy, and lasting fulfillment.

CHAPTER FIVE

Stress Reduction and Balance: Nurturing Well-Being in the Okinawan Way

Introduction: In this chapter, we will explore the strategies and techniques employed by Okinawans to manage stress and maintain balance in their lives. We will delve into the practices they embrace, such as meditation, relaxation methods, effective time management, and the cultivation of social connections. By understanding and incorporating these practices into our own lives, we can reduce stress, enhance well-being, and promote a harmonious balance.

Meditation and Mindfulness: We will begin by examining the role of meditation and mindfulness in the lives of Okinawans. We will explore the various meditation techniques they employ, such as focused attention, loving-kindness, and body scan meditations. We will discuss the benefits of regular meditation practice, including stress reduction, improved mental clarity, emotional balance, and increased self-awareness. We will also provide practical guidance on how to incorporate meditation into our daily routines.

Relaxation Methods: Okinawans have developed effective relaxation methods to counteract the demands of modern life. We will explore techniques such as deep breathing exercises, progressive muscle relaxation, and visualization. We will discuss the physiological and psychological benefits of relaxation, including reduced muscle tension, improved sleep quality, and enhanced stress resilience. By incorporating these relaxation methods into our lives, we can restore balance and promote overall well-being.

Effective Time Management: Time management plays a crucial role in reducing stress and achieving a sense of balance. We will explore the Okinawan approach to time management, which emphasizes a slower pace of life and the practice of "yutori" (finding space and time). We will discuss strategies for prioritizing tasks, setting boundaries, and creating a balanced schedule that allows for rest, leisure, and meaningful activities. By adopting effective time management techniques, we can reduce stress, increase productivity, and create more fulfilling lives.

The Importance of Social Connections: Okinawans recognize the value of strong social connections in promoting well-being and reducing stress. We will explore their emphasis on building and maintaining relationships with family, friends, and community. We will discuss the concept of "moai" (close-knit social support networks) and how it fosters a sense of belonging, emotional support, and resilience. We will also provide practical tips for cultivating social connections and nurturing meaningful relationships in our own lives.

Finding Balance in Work and Leisure: Achieving a healthy work-life balance is vital for stress reduction and overall well-being. We will discuss the Okinawan perspective on work and leisure, which emphasizes the importance of finding joy and purpose in both. We will explore the concept of "ikigai" (finding purpose and meaning in life) in the context of work, and how it contributes to a sense of fulfillment and balance. We will also highlight the significance of leisure activities, hobbies, and creative pursuits in rejuvenating the mind and reducing stress.

Embracing Nature and Physical Well-being: The Okinawan connection to nature and physical well-being is integral to their stress reduction practices. We will explore their appreciation for the natural environment, engaging in outdoor activities, and spending time in green spaces. We will discuss the benefits of connecting with nature, such as reduced stress levels, improved mood, and enhanced cognitive function. We will also emphasize the importance of regular physical exercise and movement in maintaining physical and mental well-being.

Conclusion: As we conclude our exploration of stress reduction and balance in the Okinawan way, we are reminded of the significance of incorporating these practices into our own lives. By embracing meditation, relaxation methods, effective time management, and nurturing social connections, we can reduce stress, restore balance, and promote overall well-being. The wisdom of Okinawans serves as a guiding light, reminding us that by cultivating

these practices, we can navigate the demands of modern life with greater ease and find a sense of harmony within ourselves and our surroundings.

In our fast-paced and often stressful world, learning from the Okinawan approach can be transformative. By incorporating meditation and mindfulness into our daily routines, we can cultivate a deeper sense of presence, calm, and self-awareness. Engaging in relaxation methods such as deep breathing exercises and visualization allows us to release tension, promote relaxation, and recharge our energy.

Effective time management is key to reducing stress and achieving balance. By setting priorities, creating boundaries, and allowing ourselves ample time for rest and rejuvenation, we can create a more harmonious and fulfilling life. Balancing work and leisure, and finding joy and purpose in both, enables us to nurture our well-being and find fulfillment in our daily activities.

The importance of social connections cannot be overstated. By fostering meaningful relationships, building supportive networks, and nurturing a sense of belonging, we create a strong support system that buffers against stress and enhances our overall well-being. Embracing the Okinawan concept of "moai" encourages us to invest in our relationships and create a sense of community.

Connecting with nature and prioritizing physical well-being are vital aspects of stress reduction and balance. Spending time in nature, whether through outdoor activities or simply immersing ourselves in its beauty, allows us to find solace, renew our energy, and gain perspective. Regular physical exercise, tailored to our abilities and preferences, supports our physical health and enhances our mental well-being.

As we integrate these practices into our lives, it is important to remember that the journey toward stress reduction and balance is a personal one. Each individual's needs and preferences may differ, and it is essential to listen to our own bodies and inner wisdom. By embracing the wisdom of the Okinawan people and adapting these practices to our own contexts, we can cultivate a life of greater peace, fulfillment, and well-being.

Incorporating the strategies and techniques employed by Okinawans to manage stress and maintain balance is a powerful step towards nurturing our well-being. By embracing meditation, relaxation methods, effective time management, the importance of social connections, and the harmony of nature and physical well-being, we can create a more balanced and fulfilling life. Let us embark on this journey with an open mind and a willingness to prioritize our own well-being, knowing that in doing so, we contribute to a more harmonious and balanced world.

CHAPTER SIX

Nature's Healing Power: Discovering the Bond between Okinawans and their Natural Environment

Introduction: In this chapter, we delve into the profound connection between Okinawans and their natural environment, and how it contributes to their well-being and longevity. We explore the healing power of nature, the therapeutic benefits of Okinawa's green spaces, and the profound impact of the ocean on physical and mental health. By understanding and embracing the relationship between humans and nature, we can tap into its healing potential and enhance our own well-being.

The Therapeutic Benefits of Nature: We begin by examining the therapeutic benefits of spending time in nature. We explore the calming effect of natural environments on the mind and body, and the restorative power of being surrounded by greenery, fresh air, and natural sounds. We discuss the research-backed benefits of nature exposure, including stress reduction, improved mood, enhanced cognitive function, and increased vitality. By immersing ourselves in nature, we can experience its profound healing effects.

Okinawa's Green Spaces: Okinawa is blessed with abundant green spaces, including lush forests, botanical gardens, and picturesque parks. We delve into the unique features of Okinawa's natural landscapes and their significance in promoting well-being. We explore the concept of "forest bathing" and the practice of Shinrin-yoku, which involves immersing oneself in the healing atmosphere of the forest. We also highlight specific green spaces in Okinawa known for their therapeutic qualities and share practical tips for connecting with nature in our own surroundings.

The Ocean's Impact on Health: The ocean holds a special place in the hearts of Okinawans, and its proximity has a profound impact on their physical and mental health. We explore the therapeutic benefits of the ocean, including the calming sound of waves, the soothing effect of coastal breezes, and the positive impact of negative ions present near the shoreline. We discuss the Okinawan tradition of "uminchu" (ocean healing) and how activities such as swimming, snorkeling, and simply immersing oneself in the ocean contribute to physical well-being and emotional rejuvenation.

Harnessing the Power of Nature: We provide practical guidance on how to harness the power of nature in our own lives. We discuss the benefits of outdoor activities such as hiking, gardening, and nature walks, and their role in promoting physical fitness, reducing stress, and fostering a deeper connection with the natural world. We explore the concept of biophilia, the innate human affinity for nature, and how we can incorporate elements of nature into our living spaces to create a more harmonious and healing environment.

Conservation and Sustainability: We emphasize the importance of conservation and sustainability in preserving the natural beauty of Okinawa and beyond. We discuss the Okinawan philosophy of "Yambaru," which encompasses the notion of living in harmony with nature and protecting its delicate ecosystems. We explore how our individual choices and actions can contribute to a more sustainable future, ensuring that future generations can continue to benefit from the healing power of nature.

Nature's healing power is undeniable, and Okinawans have long recognized and embraced this connection. By immersing ourselves in nature, exploring Okinawa's green spaces, and embracing the therapeutic benefits of the ocean, we can enhance our physical and mental well-being. Let us remember to cherish and protect the natural world, recognizing that in doing so, we nurture our own well-being and contribute to a more sustainable and harmonious future.

Exploring Okinawan Traditions in Nature: In this section, we delve deeper into the specific traditions and practices of Okinawans that demonstrate their profound connection with nature. We explore rituals and ceremonies that honor the natural elements, such as the appreciation of cherry blossoms in spring and the celebration of the harvest season. We also delve into the art of tea ceremonies held in serene garden settings, where participants engage in mindfulness and appreciation of nature's beauty. By understanding and embracing these traditions, we can gain insight into

Okinawan culture and deepen our own connection with the natural world.

Healing Gardens and Botanical Medicine: Okinawa is home to a rich variety of plants and botanical treasures that have been utilized for centuries for their healing properties. We explore the concept of healing gardens, where specific plants are intentionally cultivated to promote physical and mental well-being. We discuss the therapeutic uses of native Okinawan plants, such as turmeric, goya (bitter melon), and mugwort, and how they are incorporated into traditional medicine and dietary practices. By appreciating the power of botanical medicine, we can explore natural remedies and incorporate them into our own wellness routines.

Environmental Stewardship and Eco-Tourism: Okinawans have a deep respect for their natural environment and are committed to its preservation. We delve into the initiatives and practices that promote environmental stewardship and sustainable living on the island. We explore the concept of eco-tourism and how it provides opportunities for visitors to experience and appreciate Okinawa's natural wonders while supporting conservation efforts. By learning from Okinawan approaches to sustainable living and engaging in responsible tourism, we can contribute to the preservation of natural resources and the protection of fragile ecosystems.

Nature and Cultural Identity: The profound connection between nature and cultural identity is a fundamental aspect of Okinawan culture. We examine how nature is woven into Okinawan art, music, and storytelling, reflecting a deep reverence for the natural world. We explore traditional crafts inspired by nature, such as shellwork and weaving, which serve as a testament to the importance of nature in Okinawan artistic expressions. By appreciating the intersection of nature and cultural identity, we can deepen our understanding of Okinawan traditions and their holistic approach to well-being.

Continuing the Legacy: In the final section of this chapter, we address the importance of continuing the legacy of nature's healing power in our own lives and communities. We discuss ways to incorporate nature into our daily routines, whether through spending time in local parks, cultivating our own gardens, or engaging in outdoor activities. We also emphasize the significance of passing down the wisdom of nature's healing power to future generations, fostering an appreciation for the natural world and its role in promoting well-being and sustainability.

Conclusion: The bond between Okinawans and their natural environment is a testament to the profound healing power of nature. By exploring Okinawan traditions, healing gardens, environmental stewardship, and the cultural significance of nature, we can deepen our own connection with the natural world. Let us draw inspiration from Okinawa's profound reverence for nature, embracing its healing power and committing to its preservation. In doing so, we not only enhance our own well-being but also contribute to a more harmonious and sustainable world for generations to come.

CHAPTER SEVEN

Aging with Grace: Embracing the Wisdom of Okinawan Longevity

Introduction: In this chapter, we delve into the Okinawan perspective on aging and the wisdom passed down through generations. We explore how Okinawans approach the aging process, embrace their life stages, and maintain a positive outlook on growing older. By understanding and adopting their mindset, we can gain insights into aging gracefully and living a fulfilling life at any age.

The Value of Experience and Wisdom: We begin by discussing the Okinawan appreciation for experience and wisdom that comes with age. We explore how Okinawans view aging as a valuable stage of life, where accumulated knowledge, insights, and life lessons are treasured. We delve into the respect and reverence given to elders in Okinawan culture, highlighting the intergenerational exchange of wisdom that enriches the entire community. By embracing the value of experience and wisdom, we can shift our perspective on aging and approach it with a positive mindset.

Holistic Health and Self-Care: Okinawans prioritize holistic health and self-care throughout their lives, including as they age. We explore their approach to physical, mental, and emotional well-being, emphasizing the importance of regular exercise, nutritious diet, and stress reduction techniques. We discuss how Okinawans engage in activities such as tai chi, yoga, and gentle movement practices to maintain flexibility, balance, and overall vitality. By adopting a holistic approach to health and self-care, we can enhance our well-being and age with grace.

Sense of Purpose and Engagement: Okinawans maintain a strong sense of purpose and engagement in life, even as they age. We explore the concept of "ikigai" and how Okinawans find meaning and purpose in their daily activities. We discuss the importance of staying socially connected, pursuing hobbies and interests, and engaging in meaningful work or volunteer activities. By cultivating a sense of purpose and remaining engaged in life, we can continue to find fulfillment and joy as we age.

Resilience and Adaptability: Okinawans demonstrate remarkable resilience and adaptability in the face of life's challenges. We delve into their ability to navigate transitions and embrace change with a positive attitude. We explore the concept of "nankuru naisa" - a phrase that reflects their optimistic outlook and ability to overcome adversity. We discuss how cultivating resilience and adaptability can help us navigate the inevitable changes and transitions that come with aging, allowing us to embrace each stage of life with grace.

Community and Social Connections: Community and social connections play a vital role in the lives of Okinawans as they age. We explore the concept of "moai," close-knit social support networks that provide companionship, emotional support, and a sense of belonging. We discuss the importance of fostering and maintaining social connections as we age, whether through family, friends, or community involvement. By prioritizing community and nurturing social connections, we can enhance our well-being and age with a sense of belonging and support.

Legacy and Generational Impact: Okinawans hold a deep understanding of the impact they can have on future generations. We discuss how they embrace their role as mentors and pass down their wisdom, traditions, and values to younger generations. We explore the concept of leaving a positive legacy and the sense of purpose it brings. By recognizing the impact we can have on future generations, we can find fulfillment and purpose in contributing to the well-being of those who come after us.

Conclusion: The Okinawan perspective on aging offers valuable insights into embracing the wisdom of the years and living a fulfilling life at any age. By valuing experience and wisdom, prioritizing holistic health and self-care, cultivating a sense of purpose, resilience, and adaptability, fostering social connections, and embracing the importance of leaving a positive legacy, we can age with grace and find meaning in every stage of life.

We explore practical tips and strategies for incorporating these principles into our own lives, such as staying physically active, maintaining a healthy diet, cultivating a sense of purpose through meaningful activities, fostering social connections, and engaging in lifelong learning. We also discuss the importance of self-reflection and embracing the changes and challenges that come with aging, viewing them as opportunities for growth and personal development.

Furthermore, we delve into the importance of shifting societal attitudes towards aging and promoting a culture of respect and appreciation for the wisdom and contributions of older adults. By challenging ageist stereotypes and recognizing the valuable role that seniors play in society, we can create a more inclusive and supportive environment for people of all ages.

In conclusion, embracing the Okinawan perspective on aging allows us to approach this natural process with grace, wisdom, and a positive outlook. By valuing experience, prioritizing holistic well-being, nurturing social connections, and leaving a positive legacy, we can live fulfilling lives and inspire others to do the same. Let us embrace the wisdom of Okinawa and age with grace, making each day a celebration of life's journey.

CHAPTER EIGHT

The Okinawa Secret in Practice: Embracing the Principles of Longevity in Everyday Life

Introduction: In this chapter, we provide practical guidance on how to incorporate Okinawan principles into everyday life. We offer actionable steps, tips, and recipes to help readers adopt the Okinawa lifestyle and integrate its key elements into their own routines. By implementing these practices, we can enhance our well-being, promote longevity, and embrace a more balanced and fulfilling life.

Creating a Balanced Plate: We begin by exploring the Okinawan diet in greater detail and providing practical tips for creating a balanced plate inspired by their culinary traditions. We discuss the importance of including a variety of colorful fruits and vegetables, whole grains, lean proteins, and healthy fats in our meals. We provide recipe ideas that showcase Okinawan ingredients and flavors, offering options for breakfast, lunch, dinner, and snacks that reflect the principles of the Okinawan diet.

Mindful Eating Practices: Mindful eating is a key component of the Okinawan lifestyle. We delve into the practice of savoring each bite, being present in the moment, and paying attention to hunger and fullness cues. We offer tips for practicing mindful eating, such as slowing down during meals, minimizing distractions, and engaging all the senses while enjoying food. By adopting mindful eating practices, we can develop a healthier relationship with food and derive greater satisfaction from our meals.

Incorporating Physical Activity: Physical activity plays a crucial role in the Okinawan lifestyle. We discuss the importance of regular exercise for maintaining overall health and vitality. We explore Okinawan activities such as tai chi, yoga, and walking, which promote strength, flexibility, and balance. We provide practical suggestions for incorporating physical activity into daily routines, including tips for setting achievable goals, finding enjoyable forms of exercise, and staying motivated.

Cultivating a Sense of Purpose: Discovering and nurturing a sense of purpose is a fundamental aspect of the Okinawan way of life. We offer guidance on identifying personal passions, interests, and values, and finding activities that align with our individual sense of purpose. We explore practical steps for setting goals, pursuing meaningful work or hobbies, and finding fulfillment in everyday life. By cultivating a sense of purpose, we can experience greater joy and satisfaction in our daily endeavors.

Stress Reduction and Self-Care: Managing stress is vital for overall well-being, and Okinawans have developed effective strategies for stress reduction. We discuss various techniques such as meditation, deep breathing exercises, and engaging in relaxation activities like spending time in nature or enjoying a warm bath. We emphasize the importance of self-care and offer practical suggestions for incorporating self-care practices into daily routines, including setting boundaries, prioritizing restful sleep, and engaging in activities that bring joy and rejuvenation.

Building Social Connections: Strong social connections are a cornerstone of the Okinawan lifestyle. We explore the importance of fostering meaningful relationships and building a supportive network of friends and loved ones. We provide practical tips for strengthening social connections, such as joining community groups, volunteering, and engaging in activities that promote interaction and camaraderie. By prioritizing social connections, we can experience greater happiness, a sense of belonging, and improved overall well-being.

Continuing the Journey: In the final section of this chapter, we encourage readers to continue their journey towards adopting the Okinawan principles in their lives. We provide guidance on setting realistic goals, creating a supportive environment, and celebrating progress along the way. We also emphasize the importance of self-compassion and embracing a mindset of lifelong learning and growth.

Conclusion: Incorporating the Okinawan principles into everyday life is within reach for anyone seeking a more balanced and fulfilling existence. By creating a balanced plate, practicing mindful eating, engaging in regular physical activity, cultivating a sense of purpose, managing stress through self-care, and building social connections, we can embrace the Okinawan way of life and experience its profound benefits.

In this chapter, we have provided actionable steps, practical tips, and delicious recipes to help you integrate the Okinawa lifestyle into your everyday routines. By creating balanced and nourishing meals inspired by the Okinawan diet, practicing mindful eating, and engaging in regular physical activity, you can enhance your overall well-being and promote longevity.

We have also highlighted the importance of cultivating a sense of purpose and finding activities that bring meaning and fulfillment to your life. By managing stress through various relaxation techniques and prioritizing self-care, you can maintain a healthy mind and body. Lastly, we have emphasized the significance of building and nurturing social connections, as they contribute to a sense of belonging, happiness, and overall well-being.

As you embark on this journey, remember to be patient with yourself and celebrate small victories along the way. The Okinawa lifestyle is not about perfection but rather a commitment to making positive changes that align with your values and promote a balanced and fulfilling life.

By incorporating the Okinawan principles into your daily life, you have the opportunity to experience the transformative power of this ancient wisdom. Let the Okinawa Secret guide you towards a healthier, happier, and more purposeful existence.

CHAPTER NINE

Beyond Okinawa: Applying the Okinawa Secret to Global Health and Well-being

Introduction: In this chapter, we explore the broader implications of the Okinawa secret and its relevance to global health and well-being. While Okinawa has long been recognized as a unique region with exceptional longevity, the principles that contribute to their health and vitality can be adapted and applied in different cultural contexts worldwide. We discuss how Okinawan principles can inspire individuals, communities, and societies to promote longevity, happiness, and vitality.

Cultural Adaptation: We delve into the concept of cultural adaptation, emphasizing the importance of understanding and respecting diverse cultural contexts. While the Okinawan way of life may not be directly applicable to every culture, we explore how its principles can be adapted and integrated into different lifestyles. By embracing the core values of the Okinawan secret, such as balanced nutrition, physical activity, purposeful living, stress reduction, and social connections, individuals and communities can adopt practices that align with their own cultural backgrounds.

Balancing Tradition and Modernity: We discuss the challenge of balancing tradition and modernity in today's fast-paced world. As societies undergo rapid changes, it is crucial to find ways to preserve the wisdom of traditional practices while embracing the benefits of modern advancements. We explore how Okinawa has navigated this balance, maintaining their cultural heritage while adapting to the realities of the modern era. We highlight the importance of integrating Okinawan principles into contemporary lifestyles to foster health and well-being.

Inspiring Healthier Lifestyles: The Okinawa secret serves as a powerful source of inspiration for promoting healthier lifestyles globally. We discuss how the principles of the Okinawan lifestyle can be communicated and shared through various mediums, including education, media, and community initiatives. We explore the potential for public health campaigns and policies to incorporate Okinawan principles, encouraging individuals and communities to prioritize nutrition, physical activity, purpose, stress reduction, and social connections.

Prevention and Longevity: The Okinawan secret emphasizes the importance of prevention and proactive health measures. We discuss how the principles of the Okinawan lifestyle align with the concept of preventive medicine, emphasizing the value of maintaining health and well-being throughout life. We explore how adopting Okinawan practices can help reduce the burden of chronic diseases and promote longevity on a global scale. By prioritizing preventive measures, societies can strive for healthier populations and reduced healthcare costs.

Cultivating Global Communities of Well-being: We emphasize the power of global communities in promoting well-being. By connecting individuals and communities across different cultural contexts, we can share knowledge, experiences, and best practices related to the Okinawan principles. We explore the potential for creating global communities of well-being, where individuals and organizations collaborate to support each other in adopting and adapting the Okinawan secret. We discuss the role of technology, social media, and online platforms in facilitating these connections.

The Okinawa secret transcends its geographic boundaries and offers valuable insights into promoting longevity, happiness, and vitality globally. By adapting and applying its principles in different cultural contexts, we can inspire healthier lifestyles, preserve cultural heritage, and foster well-being on a global scale. Let us embrace the lessons of Okinawa and work together towards a healthier, happier, and more vibrant world.

Sustainable Living Practices: We explore how the Okinawa secret aligns with the principles of sustainability and environmental stewardship. Okinawans have a deep respect for nature and understand the interconnectedness between their well-being and the health of the planet. We discuss how individuals and communities can adopt sustainable practices such as reducing waste, conserving energy, and supporting local agriculture. By embracing eco-friendly habits, we can not only enhance our own well-being but also contribute to the preservation of the planet for future generations.

Promoting Cultural Exchange and Learning: The Okinawa secret offers an opportunity for cultural exchange and learning. We discuss how individuals and communities from different parts of the world can engage with Okinawan culture, traditions, and practices to gain a deeper understanding of the principles behind their longevity and well-being. We explore the potential for cultural exchange programs, study tours, and collaborative projects that foster mutual learning and appreciation of diverse cultures. By embracing cultural exchange, we can broaden our perspectives and discover new approaches to health and well-being.

Challenges and Adaptation: We acknowledge the challenges that may arise when attempting to apply the Okinawa secret in different cultural contexts. Cultural, social, and economic factors may influence the feasibility and effectiveness of certain practices. We discuss the importance of adaptation, recognizing that while the core principles remain valuable, the specific methods of implementation may need to be tailored to suit local circumstances. By acknowledging these challenges and fostering an open dialogue, we can find innovative solutions and adapt the Okinawan principles to diverse cultural settings.

Research and Collaboration: We highlight the importance of research and collaboration in further understanding the Okinawa secret and its implications for global health and well-being. We discuss the need for interdisciplinary studies, involving fields such as nutrition, psychology, sociology, and public health, to gather empirical evidence and explore the effectiveness of Okinawan practices in different populations. We encourage collaboration among researchers, policymakers, and communities to share findings, exchange ideas, and collectively work towards promoting longevity, happiness, and vitality worldwide.

Conclusion: The Okinawa secret holds valuable insights that extend beyond the borders of Okinawa itself. By adapting and applying its principles in diverse cultural contexts, we can promote healthier lifestyles, preserve cultural heritage, foster sustainability, and cultivate global communities of well-being. The Okinawa secret offers an invitation to explore, learn, and collaborate, as we strive to enhance the health and well-being of individuals and societies worldwide. Let us embrace the global relevance of the Okinawa secret and work together towards a healthier, happier, and more sustainable future for all.

CHAPTER TEN

Embracing the Eternal Isle Within: The Transformative Power of the Okinawa Secret

Introduction: In this final chapter, we invite readers to reflect on the transformative power of the Okinawa secret and how it can positively impact their lives. We encourage readers to embrace the wisdom of Okinawa, make meaningful changes, and embark on a personal journey towards enhanced health, longevity, and fulfillment. By internalizing the principles of the Okinawa secret, we can cultivate a deeper connection with ourselves and experience profound transformations.

Finding Inner Balance: We explore the concept of inner balance and its significance in the Okinawan way of life. By prioritizing physical, mental, and emotional well-being, we can create a harmonious and balanced internal landscape. We discuss the importance of self-reflection, self-care, and mindfulness practices in achieving inner balance. By nurturing our inner selves, we can enhance our overall well-being and tap into our full potential.

Embracing Change and Growth: Change is an inherent part of life, and the Okinawa secret teaches us to embrace it with open arms. We discuss the importance of adapting to life's challenges, embracing new experiences, and viewing change as an opportunity for growth. We explore practical strategies for cultivating resilience and flexibility, enabling us to navigate the complexities of life with grace and courage.

Living in the Present Moment: The Okinawa secret teaches us the value of living in the present moment and savoring the beauty of each day. We delve into the practice of mindfulness and its ability to bring us closer to the essence of life. We offer guidance on incorporating mindfulness into our daily routines, cultivating gratitude, and finding joy in the simple pleasures that surround us. By living mindfully, we can experience a deeper sense of fulfillment and contentment.

Inspiring Others: We discuss the power of leading by example and inspiring others through our actions. By embracing the Okinawa secret and making positive changes in our own lives, we can become beacons of inspiration for those around us. We explore the ripple effect of our choices and behaviors, and how they can influence others to embark on their own journeys towards health, longevity, and fulfillment. By sharing our experiences and wisdom, we can create a positive impact in the lives of others.

A Lifelong Journey: We emphasize that the Okinawa secret is not a destination but a lifelong journey. It is a continuous process of growth, learning, and self-discovery. We encourage readers to remain committed to their well-being, embracing the principles of the Okinawa secret throughout their lives. We provide guidance on setting intentions, establishing supportive habits, and celebrating milestones along the way. By staying dedicated to our journey, we can unlock our full potential and create a life filled with health, joy, and purpose.

Conclusion: Embracing the eternal isle within means recognizing the transformative power of the Okinawa secret and embarking on a personal journey towards enhanced health, longevity, and fulfillment. By finding inner balance, embracing change and growth, living in the present moment, and inspiring others, we can unlock the true potential within ourselves. Let us embrace the wisdom of Okinawa, make meaningful changes, and embark on a lifelong journey towards a healthier, happier, and more purposeful life.

Final Thoughts

As we conclude this book, we want to leave you with a few final thoughts. Embracing the eternal isle within is not just about adopting the practices and principles of Okinawa; it is about embracing a mindset and way of being that can transform your life in profound ways. It is about recognizing the potential for growth, joy, and fulfillment that exists within each of us.

Remember that the journey towards health, longevity, and fulfillment is unique for everyone. It is not about striving for perfection or comparing yourself to others. Instead, it is about honoring your own path, embracing your strengths, and learning from your challenges. Embrace the process of self-discovery, and be open to the lessons and opportunities that come your way.

Stay connected to the wisdom and inspiration of Okinawa. Draw upon the lessons and practices that resonate with you, and adapt them to fit your own life and cultural context. Remember that the Okinawa secret is not confined to

Okinawa alone; it has the power to enrich lives around the world.

Lastly, cultivate a mindset of gratitude and appreciation. Take time to reflect on how far you have come and celebrate your progress. Cherish the small victories and moments of joy along the way. By cultivating gratitude, you can foster a positive outlook and attract more positivity into your life.

As you close this book, carry the spirit of Okinawa with you. Embrace the eternal isle within, and let it guide you towards a life of health, longevity, and fulfillment. May the wisdom of Okinawa continue to inspire you on your journey, and may you experience the transformative power of embracing the Okinawa secret in your own life.

Thank you for joining us on this exploration of the Okinawa secret. We wish you all the best in your pursuit of a healthier, happier, and more purposeful existence.

.....***.....